MW01147063

# Dear Alcohol,
# I'm breaking up with you.

## 90 Day Sobriety Journal For Women.

12 weeks of non-repeating, daily, guiding writing prompts, inspirational quotes, mantras and sobriety checklists to help identify triggers, change habits, get healthier, improve relationships and live a life free from hangovers.

This Journal Belongs To:

_____

Date: _____

12 Weeks of Focused non-repeating Guided Writing Prompts designed to inspire your daily journal-ing and help you to focus your thoughts, investigate your triggers & motivations, and build new, healthy habits. Each week includes a unique Mantra, Inspirational Quotes, a Wellness Check In, and a Sobriety Worksheet with helpful tips and reminders.

# Writing Prompt Categories

## Month 1: Understanding My Motivations

Week 1: My Story & Motivations

Week 2: My Sobriety Goals

Week 3: Triggers & Urges

Week 4: Gratitude & Attitude Shift

## Month 2: Healthy Mind

Week 5: Uncovering Emotional Triggers

Week 6: People In my Life: Past & Present

Week 7: Building Positive Relationships

Week 8: Letting Go of False Narratives

## Month 2: Healthy Body

Week 9:   Building New Habits

Week 10: Nourishment for My Sober Body

Week 11: Boredom, Sleep and My New Normal

Week 12: Balance, Failure & Forgiveness

# Getting Started: Check-In

Before starting your sobriety journey, lets take stock of how you are today, right now. Being honest with yourself and looking at the ugly, often embarrassing, painful truths is an important first step in your journey. Write it down... recognize it, forgive yourself... and move forward with a plan. Congratulations on taking this first step. You are amazing.

How Many days a week am I currently drinking? _____

Is alcohol interfering with the way I want to live? _____

_____

Is alcohol negatively effecting my job or ability to financially support myself? _____

_____

_____

Is alcohol negatively affecting my relationships? _____

_____

_____

_____

How long has alcohol been a negative factor in my life?

_____

Have I found myself in embarrassing situations because of my use of alcohol? _____

Do I commit to a healthy, sober, alcohol free life?

_____

I PROMISE myself to work through 90 days of journal-ing towards a sober, alcohol free life.    If I stop, mess up or have a bad day, I promise to keep going:

Signature: _____

Date: _____

# My Sobriety Tool Kit

Each sobriety journey is unique to each individual.  Some prefer group therapy... others prefer to go solo.  Some require medical intervention or rehab facilities... or simply journal-ing.  What ever it is that YOU need to have ready in your toolbox .... Gather it now.  Stock up on books and tea. Join a yoga class. Clear out the fridge. Find a therapist.  Buy cases of sparkling water...etc.  Figure out your healthy coping mechanisms that you plan to have ready to use instead of turning to alcohol.

☐ Group Meetings such as Alcoholics Anonymous

☐ Medical support including prescriptions

☐ Rehab Facility

☐ Alternative beverages such as tea, sparkling water or
   non-alcoholic beverages

☐ Exercise Classes

☐ Family Support

☐ Hot bath with essential oils

☐ An accountability partner

☐ _____

☐ _____

☐ _____

☐ _____

*Please note that for some people, quitting alcohol can be dangerous without medical support.     Please consult your physician as this journal is not meant to imply medical advice.

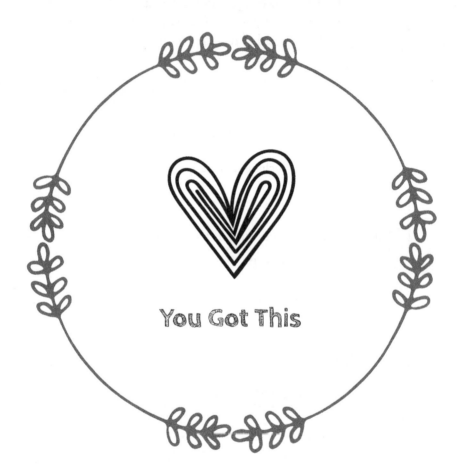

You Got This

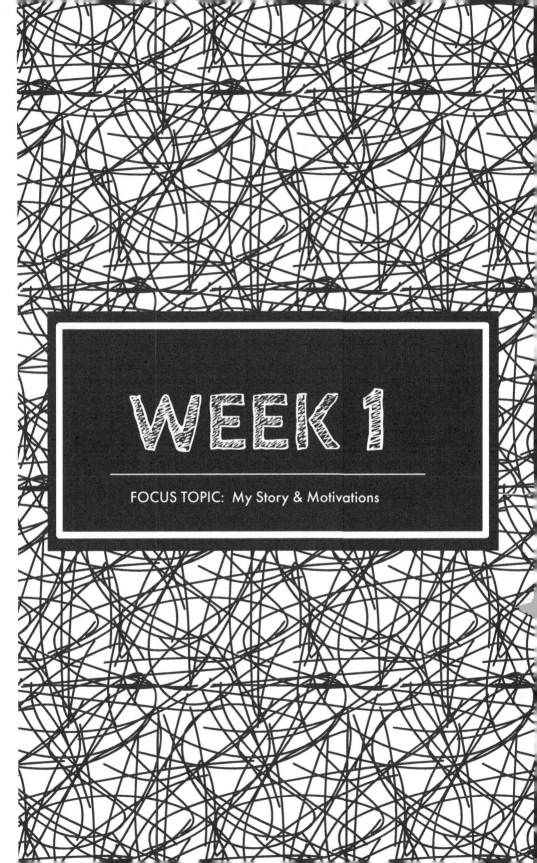

# WEEK 1

FOCUS TOPIC: My Story & Motivations

# one day one hour one minute at a time

With good reason, this often repeated phrase is used by many who are recovering from substance addictions or who are simply trying to break negative habits. Repeat this mantra to yourself all week, all day... at any moment when you are feeling weak or stressed... or if you ever feel like giving up. When you are doing dishes, driving, sitting down to order dinner, coming home from a stressful day, or walking past the alcohol aisle in the grocery store... repeat this mantra to yourself... and choose sobriety. Let the simplicity of this mantra help you through difficult moments this first week.

Date: _____ Did I stay Sober Today? | Yes | No |

My story. Describe the path that led me to the point where I
realized that I have been drinking too much alcohol. Where am
I at right now in this journey?

Date: _____ Did I stay Sober Today? | Yes | No |

What do I need in my own personal sobriety toolbox?

For example: People, books, tea, therapy, rehab, medical

support, groups....etc.  What have I tried before that I will do

differently this time?

Date: _____ Did I stay Sober Today? | Yes | No |

My own personal "rock bottom". The moment when I ultimately
knew that I absolutely needed to make changes in my life and
become sober was...

_____

_____

_____

_____

_____

_____

_____

_____

_____

_____

_____

_____

_____

_____

_____

_____

_____

_____

_____

_____

_____

_____

_____

_____

_____

_____

_____

_____

_____

_____

_____

_____

_____

One day, one hour, one minute at a time
Week 1

Date: _____ Did I stay Sober Today? | Yes | No |

The main reason(s) that I want/need to be sober in my life right now are...

Date: _____ Did I stay Sober Today? | Yes | No |

Who do I want to be sober for?  Is there someone in my life who

needs me to be sober?

Date: _____ Did I stay Sober Today? ☐ Yes ☐ No

What is the longest that I have ever went without drinking in the past? Why did I stop drinking then? Why did I start drinking again?

_____
_____
_____
_____
_____
_____
_____
_____
_____
_____
_____
_____
_____
_____
_____
_____
_____
_____
_____
_____
_____
_____
_____
_____
_____
_____
_____
_____
_____
_____
_____
_____

One day, one hour, one minute at a time
Week 1

Date: _____  Did I stay Sober Today?  | Yes | No |

Dear alcohol, I'm breaking up with you because:

_____

_____

_____

_____

_____

_____

_____

_____

_____

_____

_____

_____

_____

_____

_____

_____

_____

_____

_____

_____

_____

_____

_____

_____

_____

_____

_____

_____

_____

_____

_____

_____

_____

_____

_____

_____

_____

_____

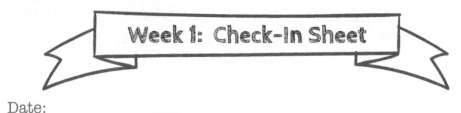

# Week 1: Check-In Sheet

Date:_____

# Days I stayed sober this week: _____

### How Does My Body Feel Today?

① ② ③ ④ ⑤ ⑥ ⑦ ⑧ ⑨ ⑩

### How is my Mood Today?

① ② ③ ④ ⑤ ⑥ ⑦ ⑧ ⑨ ⑩

Physically, I feel: _____
_____
_____
_____

Emotionally, I feel: _____
_____
_____
_____

My biggest challenges this week have been: _____
_____
_____
_____

Things I can to do to support my recovery are: _____
_____
_____

I feel proud of myself because: _____
_____
_____

Things that I can try to do a bit better next week: _____
_____

### My Top 5 Short Term Sobriety Goals

Keep it Simple and attainable. For example: take a shower, meditate for 3 minutes, tell a friend about my journey...etc.

---

---

---

---

---

### My Top 5 Long Term Sobriety Goals

Think about one month, one year, five years... What long term goals are in your heart?

---

---

---

---

---

Date:

Additional Reflections and Thoughts:

Date: _____

Additional Reflections and Thoughts: _____

_____
_____
_____
_____
_____
_____
_____
_____
_____
_____
_____
_____
_____
_____
_____
_____
_____
_____
_____
_____
_____
_____
_____
_____
_____
_____
_____
_____
_____
_____
_____
_____
_____
_____
_____

"When I got sober, I thought giving up was saying goodbye to all the fun and all the sparkle, and it turned out to be just the opposite.  That's when the SPARKLE started for me."

-MARY KARR

American Poet

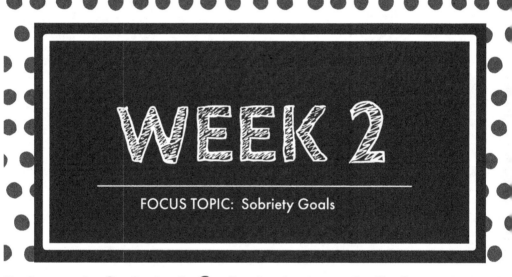

# WEEK 2

FOCUS TOPIC: Sobriety Goals

# I believe In my path I believe in myself

In the first few weeks of your sobriety journey, it is important that you empower yourself with positive messages. Even if you don't quite believe the words at first and it feels silly to say them out loud, repeating this mantra to yourself daily will help your stubborn brain to begin to believe. Trust yourself.

Use this mantra to guide your thoughts and focus your mind when you are feeling insecure about your strength of conviction. You have it in you. You can do it.

Date: _____ Did I stay Sober Today? | Yes | No |

Delve deeper into your short term goals for sobriety. Give yourself easy, simple, achievable goals. What do you hope to accomplish today in your journey to sobriety? This week?

Date: _____ Did I stay Sober Today? | Yes | No |

Delve into your long term goals?  What things do you hope to achieve that may have been out of reach before because of alcohol?

Date: _____ Did I stay Sober Today? | Yes | No |

What are some things that I can do today, in the next week and
in the years to come to replace drinking in my life?

Date: _____ Did I stay Sober Today?  [ Yes ] [ No ]

What things has drinking prevented me from accomplishing?
Think about your career, health, relationships...etc.

I believe in my path.  I believe in myself.
Week 2

Date: _____ Did I stay Sober Today? | Yes | No |

Where will I be in 5 years if I don't do anything to stop alcohol from disrupting my life?

_____

_____

_____

_____

_____

_____

_____

_____

_____

_____

_____

_____

_____

_____

_____

_____

_____

_____

_____

_____

_____

_____

_____

_____

_____

_____

_____

_____

_____

_____

_____

_____

_____

_____

I believe in my path. I believe in myself.
Week 2

Date: _____ Did I stay Sober Today? [ Yes ] [ No ]

The most important things that I want to regain during my
journey to sobriety are:

_____
_____
_____
_____
_____
_____
_____
_____
_____
_____
_____
_____
_____
_____
_____
_____
_____
_____
_____
_____
_____
_____
_____
_____
_____
_____
_____
_____
_____
_____
_____
_____
_____
_____

I believe in my path. I believe in myself.
Week 2

Date: _____ Did I stay Sober Today? | Yes | No |

Write a letter to yourself in the past and tell her why drinking
alcohol is not a good choice for your life.  Dear Past Self,

_____

_____

_____

_____

_____

_____

_____

_____

_____

_____

_____

_____

_____

_____

_____

_____

_____

_____

_____

_____

_____

_____

_____

_____

_____

_____

_____

_____

_____

_____

_____

_____

I believe in my path.  I believe in myself.
Week 2

# Week 2: Check-In Sheet

Date:_____

# Days I stayed sober this week: _____

### How Does My Body Feel Today?

(1) (2) (3) (4) (5) (6) (7) (8) (9) (10)

### How is my Mood Today?

(1) (2) (3) (4) (5) (6) (7) (8) (9) (10)

Physically, I feel: _____

_____

_____

_____

Emotionally, I feel: _____

_____

_____

_____

My biggest challenges this week have been: _____

_____

_____

_____

Things I can to do to support my recovery are: _____

_____

_____

I feel proud of myself because: _____

_____

_____

Things that I can try to do a bit better next week: _____

_____

## My Top 5 Reasons to Choose Sobriety

---

---

---

---

---

## My Top 5 Thing I'm proud of This Week

---

---

---

---

---

Date:

Additional Reflections and Thoughts:

Date: _____

Additional Reflections and Thoughts:

_____
_____
_____
_____
_____
_____
_____
_____
_____
_____
_____
_____
_____
_____
_____
_____
_____
_____
_____
_____
_____
_____
_____
_____
_____
_____
_____
_____
_____
_____
_____
_____
_____
_____
_____

"It does not matter how slowly you go, only that you  DO NOT STOP."

-CONFUCIUS

Chinese Philosopher

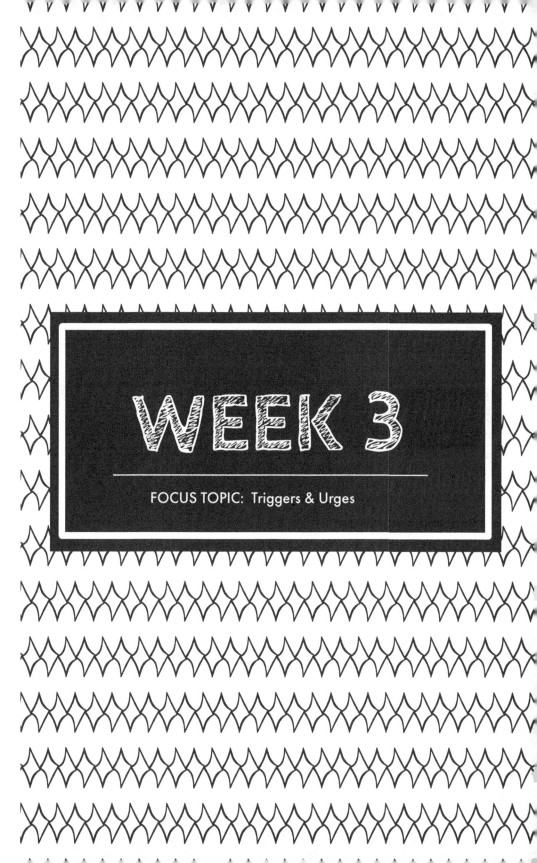

# WEEK 3

FOCUS TOPIC: Triggers & Urges

# I must reveal it to heal it

Whether we are digging in deep to reveal truths hidden to ourselves... or sharing with our loved ones the fact that our drinking has gone past the point where it is fun and controllable, we must own our journey and be proud of it. Repeat this mantra throughout the day this week. Say it out loud. Say it when you feel stressed and when you feel the urge to reach for alcohol. Instead, dig into your feelings and try to uncover the emotions that you have been covering with alcohol. When this gets uncomfortable and the emotions feel raw, be grateful for them and know that you are on the right path to healing.

Date: _____ Did I stay Sober Today? | Yes | No |

Think about the moments when I have turned to alcohol. Was I
trying to suppress emotions? What feelings did I have?    What
was happening in my life?

Date: _____ Did I stay Sober Today?  | Yes | No |

What are the events or social situations that have been
negative triggers for me? lately and how did I react? Define 3
other ways to cope that I can try next time.

_____
_____
_____
_____
_____
_____
_____
_____
_____
_____
_____
_____
_____
_____
_____
_____
_____
_____
_____
_____
_____
_____
_____
_____
_____
_____
_____
_____
_____
_____
_____
_____
_____
_____
_____

I must reveal it to heal it
Week 3

Date: _____ Did I stay Sober Today? | Yes | No |

If I had to narrow my biggest trigger down to one word, what OR
who would it be and why?

_____
_____
_____
_____
_____
_____
_____
_____
_____
_____
_____
_____
_____
_____
_____
_____
_____
_____
_____
_____
_____
_____
_____
_____
_____
_____
_____
_____
_____
_____
_____
_____
_____
_____
_____

I must reveal it to heal it
Week 3

Date: _____ Did I stay Sober Today? ☐ Yes ☐ No

How has alcohol held me back from living my best life? How
much time have I spent drinking and does it get into the way
of my dreams?

_____
_____
_____
_____
_____
_____
_____
_____
_____
_____
_____
_____
_____
_____
_____
_____
_____
_____
_____
_____
_____
_____
_____
_____
_____
_____
_____
_____
_____
_____
_____
_____
_____

I must reveal it to heal it
Week 3

Date: _____ Did I stay Sober Today? | Yes | No |

What new coping skills can I develop and use other than drinking? Write your action plan.

_____

_____

_____

_____

_____

_____

_____

_____

_____

_____

_____

_____

_____

_____

_____

_____

_____

_____

_____

_____

_____

_____

_____

_____

_____

_____

_____

_____

_____

_____

_____

_____

_____

Date: _____ Did I stay Sober Today? | Yes | No |

Do I think of drinking is a reward?    If so, how did I come
this conclusion?    Has this belief changed over time?

Date: _____ Did I stay Sober Today? | Yes | No |

How have I been using drinking to cope with situations in life?
Have I noticed that I turn to alcohol when I see the news, or
have a rough day with my family, or have a hard day at work?
What can I do to cope instead?

_____
_____
_____
_____
_____
_____
_____
_____
_____
_____
_____
_____
_____
_____
_____
_____
_____
_____
_____
_____
_____
_____
_____
_____
_____
_____
_____
_____
_____

# Week 3: Check-In Sheet

Date:_____

\# Days I stayed sober this week: _____

How Does My Body Feel Today?

① ② ③ ④ ⑤ ⑥ ⑦ ⑧ ⑨ ⑩

How is my Mood Today?

① ② ③ ④ ⑤ ⑥ ⑦ ⑧ ⑨ ⑩

Physically, I feel: _____
_____
_____
_____

Emotionally, I feel: _____
_____
_____
_____

My biggest challenges this week have been: _____
_____
_____
_____

Things I can to do to support my recovery are: _____
_____
_____

I feel proud of myself because: _____
_____
_____

Things that I can try to do a bit better next week: _____
_____

## My Primary Emotional or Social Triggers

---

---

---

---

---

## List 5 Ways to Cope with My Triggers other than Alcohol

---

---

---

---

---

Date:

Additional Reflections and Thoughts:

Date: _____
Additional Reflections and Thoughts: _____

"I wanted a drink {because} I didn't want to
feel what I was feeling, and a voice within
was telling me that I needed a drink, that I
couldn't bear it without it.  But that voice is a
LIAR.  You can always bear the pain.  It'll
hurt, it'll burn like acid in an open wound,
but you can stand it.  And, as long as you can
make yourself go on choosing the pain over
the relief,.. YOU CAN KEEP GOING."

-LAWRENCE BLOCK

Author of *Out on the Cutting Edge*

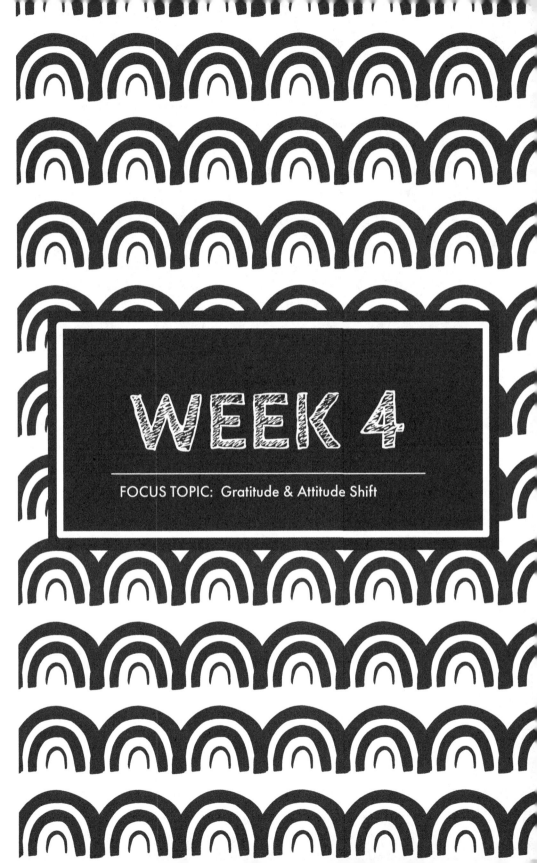

# WEEK 4

FOCUS TOPIC: Gratitude & Attitude Shift

# I am grateful for this season of change

This mantra helps us express gratitude for the opportunity to change, thrive and create what we want to see in our lives. For change to occur, we have to accept our journey, our past and forgive ourselves for our mistakes. Be grateful for the opportunity to learn and grow.

Repeat this mantra to yourself when your inner voice starts to look back on your past mistakes. Say it out loud. Forgive yourself. Love yourself. Let yourself grow and learn. Be grateful for this season of change.

Date: _____ Did I stay Sober Today? [ Yes ] [ No ]

What am I grateful for today?

I am grateful for this season of change ♡
Week 4

Date: _____ Did I stay Sober Today? | Yes | No |

What are you most proud of yourself for today? (It could be a seemingly tiny accomplishment such as a moment of self care or simply being present for someone. )

_____
_____
_____
_____
_____
_____
_____
_____
_____
_____
_____
_____
_____
_____
_____
_____
_____
_____
_____
_____
_____
_____
_____
_____
_____
_____
_____
_____
_____
_____
_____
_____
_____

Date: _____ Did I stay Sober Today? | Yes | No |

What values and hopes have I held onto in the darkest times?

Describe how these hopes and beliefs are still driving you today?

Date: _____ Did I stay Sober Today? [Yes] [No]

What are some of the simple things that give you happiness?

Is it a favorite view from a window, a person, a job, a pet?

_____
_____
_____
_____
_____
_____
_____
_____
_____
_____
_____
_____
_____
_____
_____
_____
_____
_____
_____
_____
_____
_____
_____
_____
_____
_____
_____
_____
_____
_____
_____
_____
_____
_____

I am grateful for this season of change in my
Week 4

Date: _____ Did I stay Sober Today? | Yes | No |

What am I happy about today? Or what fills my soul? How can
I hold onto this feeling in dark times?

_____
_____
_____
_____
_____
_____
_____
_____
_____
_____
_____
_____
_____
_____
_____
_____
_____
_____
_____
_____
_____
_____
_____
_____
_____
_____
_____
_____
_____
_____
_____
_____
_____
_____
_____
_____
_____

Date: _____ Did I stay Sober Today? | Yes | No |

Being on a journey towards sobriety and personal health is something to be proud of and grateful for. Have any changes happened that you are grateful for? Any lessons learned?

Date: _____     Did I stay Sober Today?  | Yes | No |

Write about a time when I was truly happy. Who was in my life?
What was I doing?  Write about a happy day in the future that
hasn't happened yet.  Then write down something I can do to
take steps towards making that day a reality.

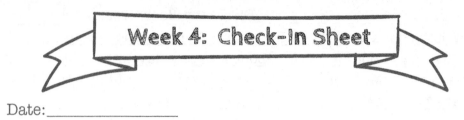

# Week 4: Check-In Sheet

Date:_____

# Days I stayed sober this week: _____

### How Does My Body Feel Today?

(1) (2) (3) (4) (5) (6) (7) (8) (9) (10)

### How is my Mood Today?

(1) (2) (3) (4) (5) (6) (7) (8) (9) (10)

Physically, I feel: _____
_____
_____
_____

Emotionally, I feel: _____
_____
_____
_____

My biggest challenges this week have been: _____
_____
_____
_____

Things I can to do to support my recovery are: _____
_____
_____

I feel proud of myself because: _____
_____
_____

Things that I can try to do a bit better next week: _____
_____

## 5 Things that I Am Grateful For In My Life

•————————————————————•

•————————————————————•

•————————————————————•

•————————————————————•

•————————————————————•

## 5 Positive Changes That I Notice About Myself When I'm Not Drinking

•————————————————————•

•————————————————————•

•————————————————————•

•————————————————————•

•————————————————————•

Date:

Additional Reflections and Thoughts:

Date: _____
Additional Reflections and Thoughts: _____

_____
_____
_____
_____
_____
_____
_____
_____
_____
_____
_____
_____
_____
_____
_____
_____
_____
_____
_____
_____
_____
_____
_____
_____
_____
_____
_____
_____
_____
_____
_____
_____
_____
_____
_____
_____
_____
_____

"Somebody once asked me how I define sobriety, and my response was 'liberation from dependence'."

-LESLIE JAMISON

Author of *The Gin Closet*

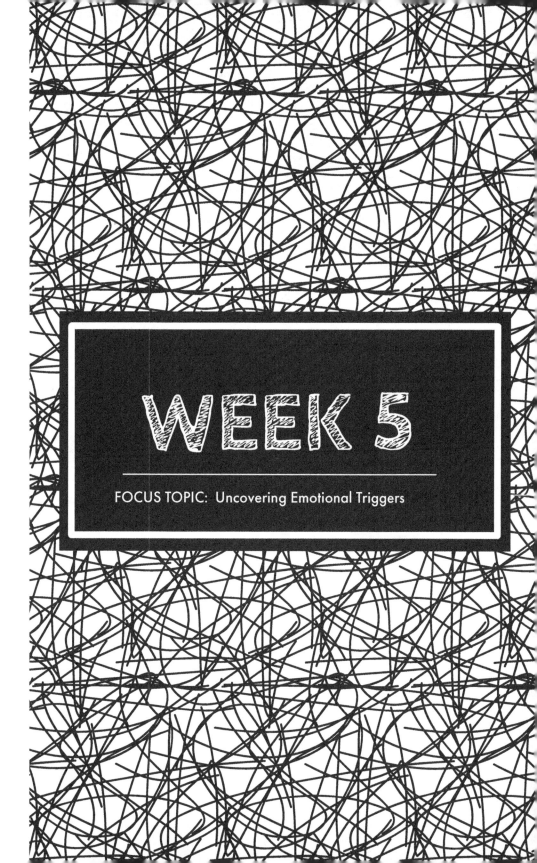

# WEEK 5

FOCUS TOPIC: Uncovering Emotional Triggers

# Sobriety is Self Love

The concept of self love is often difficult for us to grasp. We know we need to be good to others, to our kids, to our friends. But being good to ourselves is often last on the list. Self love is about making choices for our health, happiness and well being. Self love is about choosing not to abuse our bodies. Self love is about taking care of our bodies and treating ourselves with kindness and forgiveness. We must first learn how to love ourselves before we can love others. This mantra is an important defining mantra of sobriety. Repeat it daily.

Date: _____ Did I stay Sober Today? | Yes | No |

What are some of the weaknesses that you have struggled
with? If your best friend was struggling with these
weaknesses, what would you tell her? What is it that you need
to hear? Be your best friend today.

Date: _____ Did I stay Sober Today? [ Yes ] [ No ]

We are often our own bullies.   What negative self-talk do you find yourself engaging in? Write it down. Identify it. Then tell your bully to stop.

Date: _____   Did I stay Sober Today?   | Yes | No |

We often have regrets about things we have said or did when
substances were involved. Take responsibility and forgive
yourself. You can do both. Write down the things you are
going to forgive yourself for today. Then turn the page and
move forward with power and light.

Date: _____ Did I stay Sober Today? | Yes | No

Take a moment today reflect on what you are proud of yourself for. What is unique and special about you? If you're feeling empty, that's OK. What do you admire about others that you can "borrow" and incorporate into your mood, daily habits or goals?

Date: _____  Did I stay Sober Today?  | Yes | No |

Self-care can simply be scheduling a few minutes to do
something that makes you feel good about yourself.  It could be
reading a "trashy" novel, organizing a closet, scheduling a
haircut, or making a meal from scratch. What are a few things
that you can do this week?

Date: _____ Did I stay Sober Today? ☐ Yes ☐ No

Meditate for a few minutes on the stresses, thoughts, emotions, or burdens pressing into your thoughts today. Which of those can you simply let go as negative talk? Which do you need to address?

_____
_____
_____
_____
_____
_____
_____
_____
_____
_____
_____
_____
_____
_____
_____
_____
_____
_____
_____
_____
_____
_____
_____
_____
_____
_____
_____
_____
_____
_____
_____
_____
_____

Date: _____ Did I stay Sober Today? | Yes | No |

How do you respond when others compliment you? Do you
accept the compliment or reject it? Write down the good things
that others have said about you.

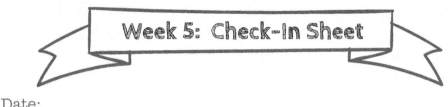

# Week 5: Check-In Sheet

Date:_____

\# Days I stayed sober this week: _____

How Does My Body Feel Today?

(1) (2) (3) (4) (5) (6) (7) (8) (9) (10)

How is my Mood Today?

(1) (2) (3) (4) (5) (6) (7) (8) (9) (10)

Physically, I feel: _____
_____
_____
_____

Emotionally, I feel: _____
_____
_____
_____

My biggest challenges this week have been: _____
_____
_____
_____

Things I can to do to support my recovery are: _____
_____
_____

I feel proud of myself because: _____
_____
_____

Things that I can try to do a bit better next week: _____
_____

## List 5 Patterns in your Life that Sabotage Your Happiness.

●———————————————————————●

●———————————————————————●

●———————————————————————●

●———————————————————————●

●———————————————————————●

## List 5 Strategies For Choosing Self Love Instead of Self Sabotage

●———————————————————————●

●———————————————————————●

●———————————————————————●

●———————————————————————●

●———————————————————————●

Date:

Additional Reflections and Thoughts:

Date: _____

Additional Reflections and Thoughts:

"Being in recovery has given me EVERYTHING of VALUE that I have in my life.  Integrity, honesty, fearlessness, faith, a relationship with God, and most of all ... GRATITUDE.  It's given me a beautiful family and an amazing career.  I'm under no illusions where I would be without the gift of alcoholism and the chance to recover from it."

-ROB LOWE

American Actor

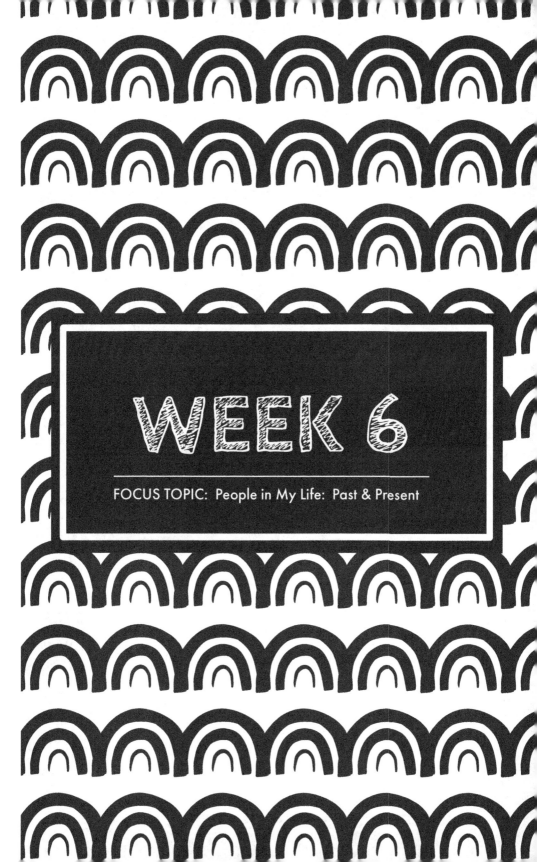

# WEEK 6

FOCUS TOPIC: People in My Life: Past & Present

# I am
# healing

Sometimes mantras don't FEEL true when we say them to ourselves. They feel artificial an we want to reject them. That is OK. That is NORMAL to feel that way. We need to say them again and again until they start to take root in our souls and become a little bit true. As time goes by, they become more true. Sobriety is a journey of healing that takes place over time. Embrace the concept that healing your body and mind from the damage that alcohol has done takes time. Repeat the mantra until you feel it.

Date: _____ Did I stay Sober Today? | Yes | No |

How have the relationships in my life impacted my sobriety positively or negatively?

Date: _____ Did I stay Sober Today? | Yes | No |

What relationships in my life have been damaged by my use of alcohol? How can I learn from those occasions? What can I do differently to improve the relationships in my life now?

I am healing
Week 6

Date: _____ Did I stay Sober Today? | Yes | No |

Who or what has been my biggest support in my journey to recovery? If my network is too small, who can I reach out to in order to build my network of support?

_____

_____

_____

_____

_____

_____

_____

_____

_____

_____

_____

_____

_____

_____

_____

_____

_____

_____

_____

_____

_____

_____

_____

_____

_____

_____

_____

_____

_____

_____

_____

_____

_____

_____

Date: _____ Did I stay Sober Today? | Yes | No |

Who/what has been my biggest adversary in my recovery?
How can I flip this story into becoming a positive learning
lesson for me? Name one reason that I am grateful for the
lessons my adversaries have taught me.

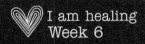

I am healing
Week 6

Date: _____ Did I stay Sober Today? | Yes | No |

Do I need others to do to help me achieve sobriety... and have I
asked for that help?

_____
_____
_____
_____
_____
_____
_____
_____
_____
_____
_____
_____
_____
_____
_____
_____
_____
_____
_____
_____
_____
_____
_____
_____
_____
_____
_____
_____
_____
_____
_____
_____
_____
_____

Date: _____ Did I stay Sober Today? | Yes | No |

Who can I call when I need to hear a friendly voice?
Why? Is there anyone that I need to take a break
from for a while? Why?

Date: _____ Did I stay Sober Today? | Yes | No |

Healing the body is part of healing the soul. Do you feel any
shifts in your body this week? What is your body telling you
that it needs? More sleep, water, exercise?

_____
_____
_____
_____
_____
_____
_____
_____
_____
_____
_____
_____
_____
_____
_____
_____
_____
_____
_____
_____
_____
_____
_____
_____
_____
_____
_____
_____
_____
_____
_____

I am healing
Week 6

# Week 6: Check-In Sheet

Date:_____

# Days I stayed sober this week: _____

### How Does My Body Feel Today?

( 1 ) ( 2 ) ( 3 ) ( 4 ) ( 5 ) ( 6 ) ( 7 ) ( 8 ) ( 9 ) ( 10 )

### How is my Mood Today?

( 1 ) ( 2 ) ( 3 ) ( 4 ) ( 5 ) ( 6 ) ( 7 ) ( 8 ) ( 9 ) ( 10 )

Physically, I feel: _____
_____
_____
_____

Emotionally, I feel: _____
_____
_____
_____

My biggest challenges this week have been: _____
_____
_____
_____

Things I can to do to support my recovery are: _____
_____
_____

I feel proud of myself because: _____
_____
_____

Things that I can try to do a bit better next week: _____
_____

## 5 Relationships In My Life That Are Effected By My Drinking/Sobriety

- ●————————————————●
- ●————————————————●
- ●————————————————●
- ●————————————————●
- ●————————————————●

## List 5 Social Situations Where Alcohol is a Factor.

- ●————————————————●
- ●————————————————●
- ●————————————————●
- ●————————————————●
- ●————————————————●

Date: _____

Additional Reflections and Thoughts:

_____
_____
_____
_____
_____
_____
_____
_____
_____
_____
_____
_____
_____
_____
_____
_____
_____
_____
_____
_____
_____
_____
_____
_____
_____
_____
_____
_____
_____
_____
_____
_____
_____
_____
_____
_____
_____
_____

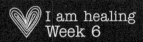

Date: _____

Additional Reflections and Thoughts: _____

"Recovery is something that you have to work on EVERY SINGLE DAY and it is something that doesn't get a day off."

-DEMI LOVATO

American Singer

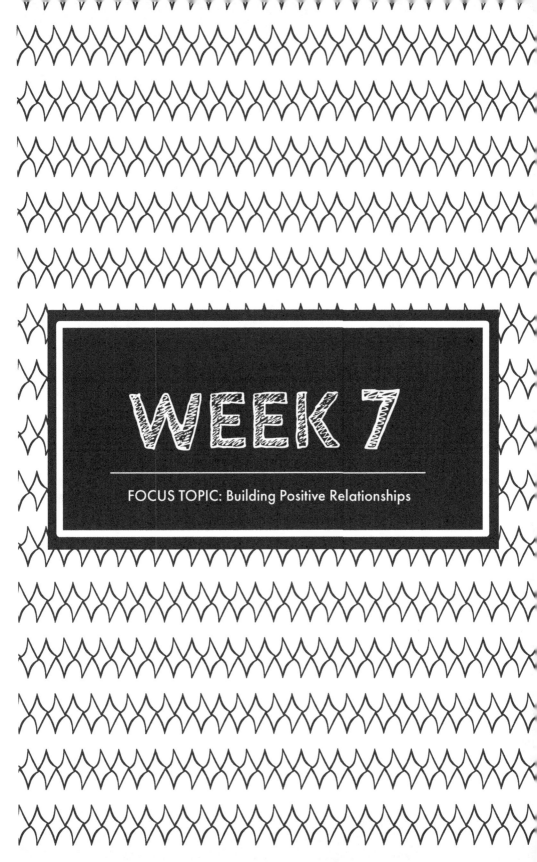

# WEEK 7

FOCUS TOPIC: Building Positive Relationships

# grow through what you go through

This often used mantra is wonderful for reminding yourself that you are growing through this process. Even if you feel defeated sometimes or make mistakes and start over, you are learning and growing. Life in sobriety has challenges that you may be experiencing now. However, if you keep reminding yourself that you are making progress and learning from this journey .... Then you can remind yourself why you started in the first place.

Repeat this mantra daily, sing it, say it, own it. When times are tough, know that you are growing.

Date: _____ Did I stay Sober Today? | Yes | No |

Dear drunk me, I forgive you for the things you did.

However, I know that growth means taking responsibility for my

actions.  Is there anyone that I need to apologize to?

Date: _____ Did I stay Sober Today? [Yes] [No]

How would you like to be seen by those closest to you? What
words do you want others to think of when they describe you?
Define ways that you can be that person today.

Date: _____ Did I stay Sober Today? | Yes | No |

What qualities do you believe are most important in friendships
and relationships? Are you being the friend/spouse/parent that
others around you need?   Or have you been preoccupied and
distracted due to drinking?  How can you be selfless to someone
today?   This could be simply listening without judgment or
talking about yourself.

Date: _____ Did I stay Sober Today? | Yes | No |

What have you gone through that are teaching moments that
you can grow from?  What have you learned?

_____
_____
_____
_____
_____
_____
_____
_____
_____
_____
_____
_____
_____
_____
_____
_____
_____
_____
_____
_____
_____
_____
_____
_____
_____
_____
_____
_____
_____
_____
_____
_____
_____
_____
_____

Date: _____ Did I stay Sober Today? | Yes | No |

Describe a time when you helped a friend in need.  Has anyone
helped you?

_____

_____

_____

_____

_____

_____

_____

_____

_____

_____

_____

_____

_____

_____

_____

_____

_____

_____

_____

_____

_____

_____

_____

_____

_____

_____

_____

_____

_____

_____

_____

_____

_____

_____

_____

Date: _____ Did I stay Sober Today? | Yes | No |

How satisfied are you with your social life? Do you have friends who you need to move on from? Do you need to find new ways to be social that don't involve drinking?

_____

_____

_____

_____

_____

_____

_____

_____

_____

_____

_____

_____

_____

_____

_____

_____

_____

_____

_____

_____

_____

_____

_____

_____

_____

_____

_____

_____

Date: _____ Did I stay Sober Today? | Yes | No |

How do you feel about your current relationship status?  How
can your shiny new sober self be a better partner to someone?

_____

_____

_____

_____

_____

_____

_____

_____

_____

_____

_____

_____

_____

_____

_____

_____

_____

_____

_____

_____

_____

_____

_____

_____

_____

_____

_____

_____

_____

_____

_____

_____

_____

_____

_____

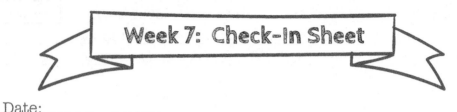

# Week 7: Check-In Sheet

Date:_____

# Days I stayed sober this week: _____

### How Does My Body Feel Today?

(1) (2) (3) (4) (5) (6) (7) (8) (9) (10)

### How is my Mood Today?

(1) (2) (3) (4) (5) (6) (7) (8) (9) (10)

Physically, I feel: _____
_____
_____
_____

Emotionally, I feel: _____
_____
_____
_____

My biggest challenges this week have been: _____
_____
_____
_____

Things I can to do to support my recovery are: _____
_____
_____

I feel proud of myself because: _____
_____
_____

Things that I can try to do a bit better next week: _____
_____

## The People in My Life Who Support My Sobriety Are:

- ●————————————————————————————————●
- ●————————————————————————————————●
- ●————————————————————————————————●
- ●————————————————————————————————●
- ●————————————————————————————————●

## 5 People Who I Can Reach Out to For Alcohol Free Lunch or Social Time

- ●————————————————————————————————●
- ●————————————————————————————————●
- ●————————————————————————————————●
- ●————————————————————————————————●
- ●————————————————————————————————●

Date:

Additional Reflections and Thoughts:

Date: _____

Additional Reflections and Thoughts: _____

_____

_____

_____

_____

_____

_____

_____

_____

_____

_____

_____

_____

_____

_____

_____

_____

_____

_____

_____

_____

_____

_____

_____

_____

_____

_____

_____

_____

_____

_____

_____

_____

_____

_____

_____

"I once heard a sober alcoholic say that drinking NEVER MADE HIM HAPPY... but it made him FEEL like he was going to be happy in about fifteen minutes. That was exactly it, and I couldn't understand why the happiness NEVER came, couldn't see that alcohol kept me trapped in a world of illusion, procrastination, paralysis. I lived always in the future... never in the present. Next time... Next time! Next time I drank it would be DIFFERENT. Next time it would make me feel good again. And all my efforts were doomed, because already drinking hadn't made me feel good in years.".

-HEATHER KING

Author of *Parched*

# WEEK 8

FOCUS TOPIC: Letting Go of False Narratives

# What YOU think of me is none of my business

Often, the moments that we have had when we were drinking have formed the opinions that others have of us. It is often difficult for them to trust our journey to sobriety. That is Ok. Forgive them. Don't try to argue. Be patient. However, their thoughts are NOT facts. They are old stories of a former you that you have left behind. You are responsible for the choices that you make from this day forward. That is all that you can do. What they think of you is none of your business. Ignore it, say thank you, and move forward with your journey.

Date: _____ Did I stay Sober Today? | Yes | No |

Are the stories that I tell myself about how great things were
when I was drinking true? Did things really happen the way
that I think they did? Were my experiences true or authentic?

Date: _____ Did I stay Sober Today? | Yes | No |

Have I ever felt that alcohol gave me courage or made me funnier or more likable? Alcohol lies to us. Define moments when alcohol tricked us into believing these false narratives.

_____
_____
_____
_____
_____
_____
_____
_____
_____
_____
_____
_____
_____
_____
_____
_____
_____
_____
_____
_____
_____
_____
_____
_____
_____
_____
_____
_____
_____
_____
_____
_____
_____
_____
_____

What you think of me is none of MY business.
Week 8

Date: _____ Did I stay Sober Today? | Yes | No |

If I were to give my past self advice about the false narratives,
that I had about alcohol, what would I tell myself?

Date: _____ Did I stay Sober Today? | Yes | No |

Where do I feel most at peace, and what can I do to bring that
sense of peace into my daily life?

_____
_____
_____
_____
_____
_____
_____
_____
_____
_____
_____
_____
_____
_____
_____
_____
_____
_____
_____
_____
_____
_____
_____
_____
_____
_____
_____
_____
_____
_____

What you think of me is none of MY business.
Week 8

Date: _____ Did I stay Sober Today? | Yes | No |

We often tell ourselves little lies such as just one drink won't hurt me....etc. Define little lies that you tell yourself. Are they true?

_____

_____

_____

_____

_____

_____

_____

_____

_____

_____

_____

_____

_____

_____

_____

_____

_____

_____

_____

_____

_____

_____

_____

_____

_____

_____

_____

_____

_____

_____

_____

_____

_____

_____

_____

What you think of me is none of MY business.
Week 8

Does society and media tell us false narratives about alcohol? If so, what are they? How do you combat the false narrative coming from those sources?

Date: _____ Did I stay Sober Today? | Yes | No |

Do my friends, family and social circle have false narratives
about alcohol?  Are they true?

# Week 8: Check-In Sheet

Date:_____

# Days I stayed sober this week: _____

How Does My Body Feel Today?

(1) (2) (3) (4) (5) (6) (7) (8) (9) (10)

How is my Mood Today?

(1) (2) (3) (4) (5) (6) (7) (8) (9) (10)

Physically, I feel: _____

_____

_____

_____

Emotionally, I feel: _____

_____

_____

_____

My biggest challenges this week have been: _____

_____

_____

_____

Things I can to do to support my recovery are: _____

_____

_____

I feel proud of myself because: _____

_____

_____

Things that I can try to do a bit better next week: _____

_____

## List 5 Lies That I Have Told Myself About Alcohol

●———————————————————————●

●———————————————————————●

●———————————————————————●

●———————————————————————●

●———————————————————————●

## List 5 False Narratives About Alcohol That Society Or Friends Have

●———————————————————————●

●———————————————————————●

●———————————————————————●

●———————————————————————●

●———————————————————————●

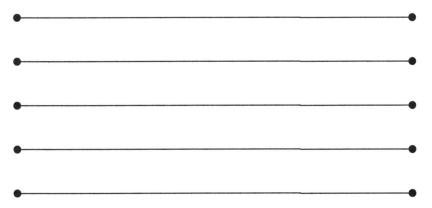

Date:

Additional Reflections and Thoughts:

Date: _____

Additional Reflections and Thoughts: _____

_____

_____

_____

_____

_____

_____

_____

_____

_____

_____

_____

_____

_____

_____

_____

_____

_____

_____

_____

_____

_____

_____

_____

_____

_____

_____

_____

_____

_____

_____

_____

_____

_____

_____

_____

_____

_____

"Drinking alcohol is like pouring gasoline on your anxiety."

-Laura McKowen

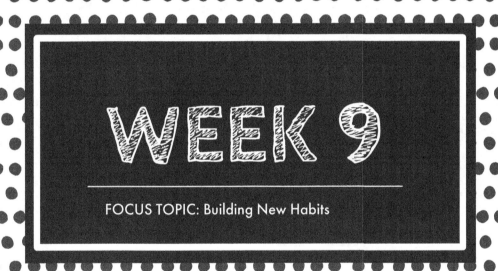

# WEEK 9

FOCUS TOPIC: Building New Habits

# nothing changes if nothing changes

This is a reminder that you have the power to make positive changes in your life by making new choices. Going back to the same old habits and patterns will only give you the same life that you had before. Small changes in your life now will have powerful effects in your future.

Repeat this mantra as you're going through your day. Use it to remind yourself to make different choices than you would have in the past.

Date: _____ Did I stay Sober Today? | Yes | No |

What is the most motivational thing I have heard or experienced
that will help me in my recovery?

Date: _____ Did I stay Sober Today? | Yes | No |

What habits do I have that have negatively impacted my sobriety?

Date: _____ Did I stay Sober Today? | Yes | No |

How can I change my daily habits to better support my sobriety?

_____
_____
_____
_____
_____
_____
_____
_____
_____
_____
_____
_____
_____
_____
_____
_____
_____
_____
_____
_____
_____
_____
_____
_____
_____
_____
_____
_____
_____
_____
_____
_____
_____
_____
_____
_____
_____

Date: _____ Did I stay Sober Today? | Yes | No |

Are you a morning person? A night person? Write about your
positive habits in your daily routine that are working for you.

_____
_____
_____
_____
_____
_____
_____
_____
_____
_____
_____
_____
_____
_____
_____
_____
_____
_____
_____
_____
_____
_____
_____
_____
_____
_____
_____
_____
_____
_____
_____
_____
_____
_____
_____

Date: _____ Did I stay Sober Today? [Yes] [No]

Think about your self dialogue. Do you have negative habits that
you need to address?

_____

_____

_____

_____

_____

_____

_____

_____

_____

_____

_____

_____

_____

_____

_____

_____

_____

_____

_____

_____

_____

_____

_____

_____

_____

_____

_____

_____

_____

_____

_____

_____

_____

Date: _____ Did I stay Sober Today? | Yes | No |

When you are in social situations, what habits do you have that negatively impact your sobriety? Or positively?

Date: _____  Did I stay Sober Today? | Yes | No |

How do you currently calm your nerves when you are feeling
stressed? What habits do you have? Are they healthy? If not,
think of new habits you can try.

_____

_____

_____

_____

_____

_____

_____

_____

_____

_____

_____

_____

_____

_____

_____

_____

_____

_____

_____

_____

_____

_____

_____

_____

_____

_____

_____

_____

_____

_____

Nothing changes if nothing changes
Week 9

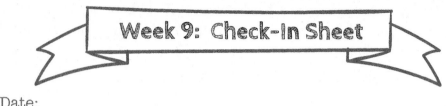

# Week 9: Check-In Sheet

Date:_____

# Days I stayed sober this week: _____

How Does My Body Feel Today?

① ② ③ ④ ⑤ ⑥ ⑦ ⑧ ⑨ ⑩

How is my Mood Today?

① ② ③ ④ ⑤ ⑥ ⑦ ⑧ ⑨ ⑩

Physically, I feel: _____
_____
_____
_____

Emotionally, I feel: _____
_____
_____
_____

My biggest challenges this week have been: _____
_____
_____
_____

Things I can to do to support my recovery are: _____
_____
_____

I feel proud of myself because: _____
_____
_____

Things that I can try to do a bit better next week: _____
_____

## Think of Tiny Daily Habits That You Can Do Every Day to Improve Your Health & Well Being

- ●—————————————————————●
- ●—————————————————————●
- ●—————————————————————●
- ●—————————————————————●
- ●—————————————————————●

## Think of 5 Habits That Are Harming You

- ●—————————————————————●
- ●—————————————————————●
- ●—————————————————————●
- ●—————————————————————●
- ●—————————————————————●

Date:

Additional Reflections and Thoughts:

Date: _____

Additional Reflections and Thoughts:

_____

_____

_____

_____

_____

_____

_____

_____

_____

_____

_____

_____

_____

_____

_____

_____

_____

_____

_____

_____

_____

_____

_____

_____

_____

_____

_____

_____

_____

_____

_____

_____

_____

_____

_____

_____

_____

"Sometimes we motivate ourselves by thinking of what we want to become. Sometimes we motivate ourselves by thinking about who we don't ever want to be again."

-Shane Niewmeyer

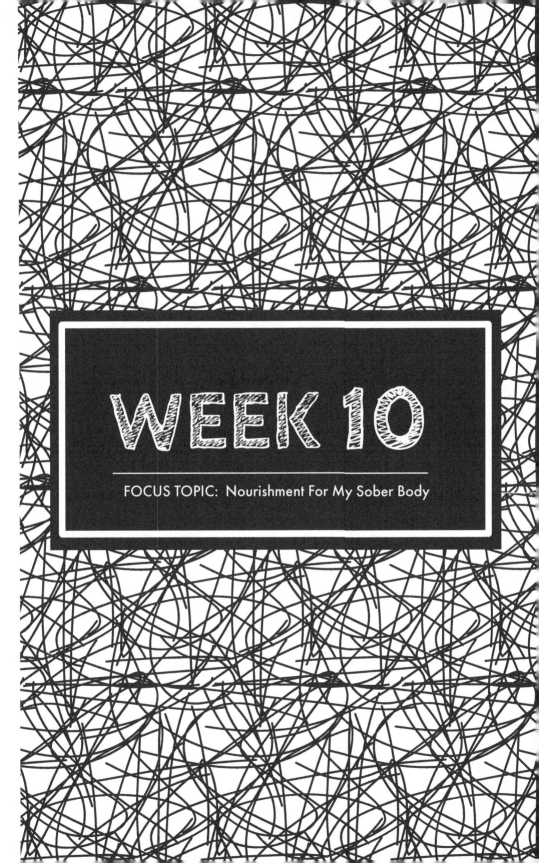

# WEEK 10

FOCUS TOPIC: Nourishment For My Sober Body

# I can do hard things ♡

Changing patterns in your life is TOUGH to do... especially when we are battling an addictive substance. But you are worthwhile. Your amazing sober life is worth the journey. You may feel negative changes physically, socially or emotionally as you move forward. You CAN handle those things. Put on your big girl pants. Wash your face. You got this.

Repeat this affirming mantra every day to remind yourself that you can do hard things.

Date: _____   Did I stay Sober Today?   | Yes | | No |

Today is so full of wonderful possibilities.   What can I do
today for my physical health and for my emotional well being?
Take a walk?  Join a gym?  Make a smoothie?  What is your
health goal today for today?  And what is your health goal in
the next few months?

Date: _____ Did I stay Sober Today? | Yes | No |

How does my body feel today?  Sit quietly, close your eyes
and pay attention to what your body is telling you.  What
nourishment do I need? What does my body need to feel
healthier?

Date: _____ Did I stay Sober Today? | Yes | No |

What changes do I feel lately in my body due to my change in
alcohol intake?  What can I do to support my sober body?

_____
_____
_____
_____
_____
_____
_____
_____
_____
_____
_____
_____
_____
_____
_____
_____
_____
_____
_____
_____
_____
_____
_____
_____
_____
_____
_____
_____
_____
_____
_____

Date: _____ Did I stay Sober Today? | Yes | No |

Have I let anything slide such as dentist appointments or health check ups? Now that I'm on a journey to sobriety, I commit to taking care of myself. Write about the way you have cared for yourself in the past.... And how you will do things differently now.

---
---
---
---
---
---
---
---
---
---
---
---
---
---
---
---
---
---
---
---
---
---
---
---
---
---
---
---
---
---
---
---
---
---
---
---

I can do hard things
Week 10

Date: _____ Did I stay Sober Today? | Yes | No |

Am I hungry, thirsty, tired? Sobriety is more of a challenge when we aren't nourishing ourselves. Have there been times in the past when you have turned to alcohol when you really needed to take care of yourself?

Date: _____ Did I stay Sober Today? | Yes | No |

Have there been any new physical feelings with my
sobriety? Are they positive or negative? Both?

Date: _____ Did I stay Sober Today? | Yes | No |

Write about how you can honor your body with a better self care
regimen. What things can you do to pamper yourself in little
ways? Or big ways? Define a new morning routine.

_____

_____

_____

_____

_____

_____

_____

_____

_____

_____

_____

_____

_____

_____

_____

_____

_____

_____

_____

_____

_____

_____

_____

_____

_____

_____

_____

_____

_____

_____

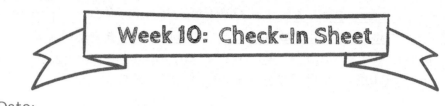

# Week 10: Check-In Sheet

Date:_____

# Days I stayed sober this week: _____

### How Does My Body Feel Today?

① ② ③ ④ ⑤ ⑥ ⑦ ⑧ ⑨ ⑩

### How is my Mood Today?

① ② ③ ④ ⑤ ⑥ ⑦ ⑧ ⑨ ⑩

Physically, I feel: _____
_____
_____
_____

Emotionally, I feel: _____
_____
_____
_____

My biggest challenges this week have been: _____
_____
_____
_____

Things I can to do to support my recovery are: _____
_____
_____

I feel proud of myself because: _____
_____
_____

Things that I can try to do a bit better next week: _____
_____

## List 5 Ways That I Can Nourish My Body Today

- _____

- _____

- _____

- _____

- _____

## List 5 Physical Habits That I Have That Hurt My Health & Sobriety

- _____

- _____

- _____

- _____

- _____

Date:

Additional Reflections and Thoughts:

Date: _____

Additional Reflections and Thoughts: _____

"...Cause sometimes you just feel tired. Feel weak, and when you feel weak, you feel like you wanna just give up. But you gotta search within you. You gotta find that inner strength. And just pull it out of you, and get that motivation to not give up, and not be a quitter, no matter how bad you wanna just fall fat on your face."

-Eminem

# WEEK 11

FOCUS TOPIC: Boredom, Sleep & My New Normal

# I have everything that I need within me

One of the biggest causes of anxiety in recovery from alcohol is that feeling that there are things we need that we don't have. We look at others who may have more resources or support and think that if we had those things, we would be fine. Comparison is the enemy of peace. Within yourself you can find: security, sensation, love, warmth, belonging, strength.

This mantra reminds us to be grateful for what we have, and to use internal resources to nourish ourselves

Date: _____ Did I stay Sober Today? | Yes | No |

Lets talk about sleep and self care.    Am I getting enough
sleep?  What else do I need to focus on to optimize my health?

_____
_____
_____
_____
_____
_____
_____
_____
_____
_____
_____
_____
_____
_____
_____
_____
_____
_____
_____
_____
_____
_____
_____
_____
_____
_____
_____
_____
_____
_____
_____

I have everything thing that I need within me
Week 11

Date: _____ Did I stay Sober Today?  [Yes] [No]

Often, people feel bored when they stop drinking. Do you find
yourself feeling bored?  What are you spending your time
doing?  What new hobbies or activities have you been hoping
to have time for in your life?

Date: _____     Did I stay Sober Today?  | Yes | No |

Do you have any new skills you want to gain, or exercise
schedules that you can try now that you have more time being
"present"?

_____
_____
_____
_____
_____
_____
_____
_____
_____
_____
_____
_____
_____
_____
_____
_____
_____
_____
_____
_____
_____
_____
_____
_____
_____
_____
_____
_____
_____
_____
_____
_____
_____
_____

I have everything I need within me ♥
Week 11

Date: _____ Did I stay Sober Today? | Yes | No |

What things have you procrastinated about that you can get done now?  Make a list.

Date: _____ Did I stay Sober Today? [Yes] [No]

Is your home clean and organized? If not, focus on how you can optimize your space to be a place of peace. Do you have obstacles to peace in your environment?

Date: _____ Did I stay Sober Today? | Yes | No |

The new sober you may be up earlier or awake later or simply staring out the window wondering what to do. Do you remember the OLD you before alcohol? Was there anything that you used to do that brought you joy?

Date: _____ Did I stay Sober Today? | Yes | No |

You have come so far in your journey?  What new things have
you accomplished lately that you couldn't have done before?
What new hopes and goals do you have with your new life of
sobriety?

_____
_____
_____
_____
_____
_____
_____
_____
_____
_____
_____
_____
_____
_____
_____
_____
_____
_____
_____
_____
_____
_____
_____
_____
_____
_____
_____
_____
_____
_____
_____

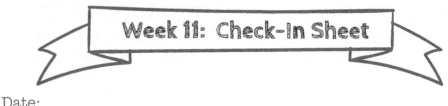

# Week 11: Check-In Sheet

Date:_____

# Days I stayed sober this week: _____

How Does My Body Feel Today?

① ② ③ ④ ⑤ ⑥ ⑦ ⑧ ⑨ ⑩

How is my Mood Today?

① ② ③ ④ ⑤ ⑥ ⑦ ⑧ ⑨ ⑩

Physically, I feel: _____
_____
_____
_____

Emotionally, I feel: _____
_____
_____
_____

My biggest challenges this week have been: _____
_____
_____
_____

Things I can to do to support my recovery are: _____
_____
_____

I feel proud of myself because: _____
_____
_____

Things that I can try to do a bit better next week: _____
_____

Think of 5 New Hobbies, Activities or Passions that You Would Like to Pursue

Think Of 5 Things That You Used to Enjoy Before Alcohol Entered Your Life

Date:

Additional Reflections and Thoughts:

Date: _____

Additional Reflections and Thoughts: _____

"I realized that I only had two choices: I was either going to die or I was going to live, and which one did I want to do? And then I said those words, 'I'll get help,' or, 'I need help. I'll get help.' And my life turned around. Ridiculous for a human being to take 16 years to say, 'I need help.'"

-SIR ELTON JOHN

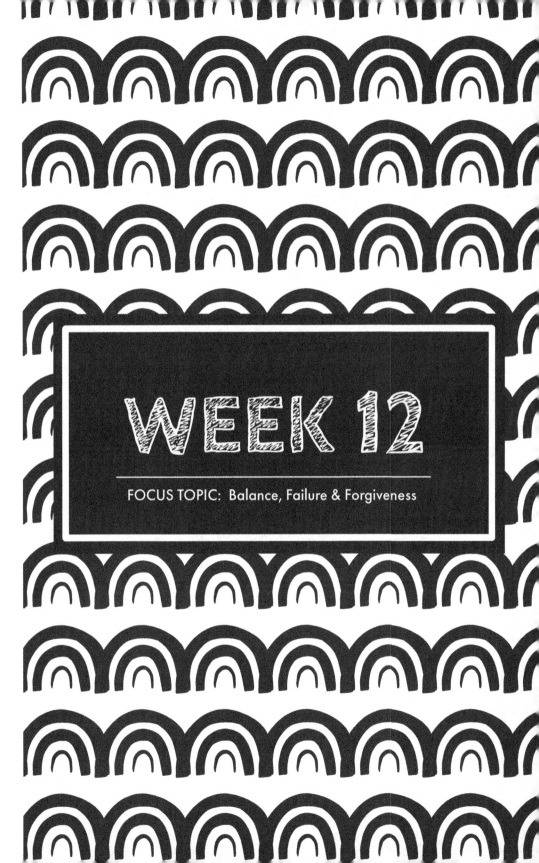

# WEEK 12

FOCUS TOPIC: Balance, Failure & Forgiveness

# PROGRESS
## not
## perfection

There are a lot of "shoulds and should nots" in sobriety. Some say there is only one way. There is only YOUR way. Sometimes, counting days that you are sober can make one feel like a failure if you go back to day one. It isn't. It is part of the journey. You are not expected to be a saint and fix everything about your life instantly. Just keep trying. Be proud of your successes and forgive yourself for your mistakes. Just keep going. Keep repeating this mantra.

Date: _____  Did I stay Sober Today?  Yes  No

In 10 years, how do I want the story of my addiction and recovery to be told?

_____
_____
_____
_____
_____
_____
_____
_____
_____
_____
_____
_____
_____
_____
_____
_____
_____
_____
_____
_____
_____
_____
_____
_____
_____
_____
_____
_____
_____
_____
_____
_____
_____

Date: _____ Did I stay Sober Today? | Yes | No |

How do I hope to one day use my sobriety to inspire others?

Do I know anyone who is struggling right now?

Date: _____ Did I stay Sober Today? | Yes | No |

In my sobriety journey, have I dropped the ball, made mistakes
and started and restarted again?  Hooray, you're normal.  Keep
on keeping on.  Define the struggles I have had on my sobriety
journey so far... and how I choose to keep going.

_____

_____

_____

_____

_____

_____

_____

_____

_____

_____

_____

_____

_____

_____

_____

_____

_____

_____

_____

_____

_____

_____

_____

_____

_____

_____

_____

_____

_____

_____

_____

Date: _____ Did I stay Sober Today? | Yes | No |

It doesn't matter how messy or imperfect your sobriety journey has been, practice self love. What things can you tell yourself to encourage yourself about past mistakes?

Date: _____ Did I stay Sober Today? | Yes | No |

Has there been anything in my sobriety journey that I'm really
proud of?

Date: _____ Did I stay Sober Today? | Yes | No |

As I move forward, how will I continue my sobriety journey? What is my game plan? Has my sobriety toolbox changed over time?

_____

_____

_____

_____

_____

_____

_____

_____

_____

_____

_____

_____

_____

_____

_____

_____

_____

_____

_____

_____

_____

_____

_____

_____

_____

_____

_____

_____

_____

_____

_____

_____

_____

_____

_____

_____

Date: _____ Did I stay Sober Today? | Yes | No |

Where am I at in my sobriety journey today, right now, in this
moment? Then make a promise to yourself to keep going, keep
trying, keep starting over if you need to.

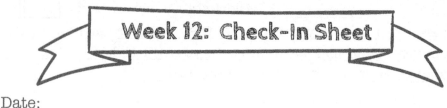

# Week 12: Check-In Sheet

Date:_____

# Days I stayed sober this week: _____

### How Does My Body Feel Today?

( 1 ) ( 2 ) ( 3 ) ( 4 ) ( 5 ) ( 6 ) ( 7 ) ( 8 ) ( 9 ) ( 10 )

### How is my Mood Today?

( 1 ) ( 2 ) ( 3 ) ( 4 ) ( 5 ) ( 6 ) ( 7 ) ( 8 ) ( 9 ) ( 10 )

Physically, I feel: _____

_____

_____

_____

Emotionally, I feel: _____

_____

_____

_____

My biggest challenges this week have been: _____

_____

_____

_____

Things I can to do to support my recovery are: _____

_____

_____

I feel proud of myself because: _____

_____

_____

Things that I can try to do a bit better next week: _____

_____

List 5 Successes That I have had in my
journey to Sobriety

●————————————————————————————————●

●————————————————————————————————●

●————————————————————————————————●

●————————————————————————————————●

●————————————————————————————————●

If I have slipped up and started over, that
is Ok.  You are still worth celebrating.
List 5 healthy rewards you can celebrate
your progress with instead of alcohol.

●————————————————————————————————●

●————————————————————————————————●

●————————————————————————————————●

●————————————————————————————————●

●————————————————————————————————●

Date: _____

Additional Reflections and Thoughts: _____

_____
_____
_____
_____
_____
_____
_____
_____
_____
_____
_____
_____
_____
_____
_____
_____
_____
_____
_____
_____
_____
_____
_____
_____
_____
_____
_____
_____
_____
_____
_____
_____
_____
_____
_____

Date: _____
Additional Reflections and Thoughts: _____

_____
_____
_____
_____
_____
_____
_____
_____
_____
_____
_____
_____
_____
_____
_____
_____
_____
_____
_____
_____
_____
_____
_____
_____
_____
_____
_____
_____
_____
_____
_____
_____
_____
_____

"In the midst of winter, I found there was, within me, an invincible summer. And that makes me happy. For it says that no matter how hard the world pushes against me, within me, there's something stronger — something better, pushing right back."

-ALBERT CAMUS

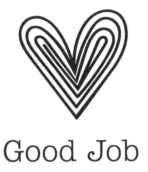

# Good Job

ArborDeco Books creates thoughtful, useful books to help you improve your life. If you see any typos or errors, please let us know. Also, we would love to hear your feedback at hello@arbordeco.com.

Also, please help us grow our small business by writing a review on Amazon!

Thank you

-ArborDeco Books

Made in the USA
Las Vegas, NV
19 January 2024

84603300R00098